Simple HCG Cookbook for Beginners

Amazingly Easy HCG Recipes for a Healthier Life

BY: Stephanie Sharp

Copyright © 2019 by Stephanie Sharp

License Notes

Copyright 2019 by Stephanie Sharp All rights reserved.

No part of this Book may be transmitted or reproduced into any format for any means without the proper permission of the Author. This includes electronic or mechanical methods, photocopying or printing.

The Reader assumes all risk when following any of the guidelines or ideas written as they are purely suggestion and for informational purposes. The Author has taken every precaution to ensure accuracy of the work but bears no responsibility if damages occur due to a misinterpretation of suggestions.

wwwwwwwwwwwwwwwwwwwwwwwww

Table of Contents

Introduction 6

    Chocolate Mousse 8

    Asian Noodle Soup 10

    Basic Egg Omelet 13

    Cucumber Slices 15

    Classic Chicken Noodle Soup 17

    Baked Apple Slices 21

    Chicken Curry Soup 23

    Savory Fish Stew 26

    Tomato Soup 29

    Summertime Spinach Salad 32

    Low-Calorie Chili 34

    HCG Approved Deviled Eggs 37

    Tokyo Cucumber Salad 40

Taco Salad 43

Grilled Chicken Salad 46

Fried Chicken Tenders 50

Shredded Barbecue Chicken Salad 53

Hard-Boiled Egg Salad 56

Beef-Stuffed Cabbage Rolls 59

Mongolian Beef Bowl 62

Tilapia del Rio 65

Applesauce 68

Scrumptious Scrambled Eggs 70

Sloppy Joes 73

Radish Chips 76

Dijon Mustard Chicken 79

Mexican Egg Omelet 82

HCG Approved Crab Cakes 85

Spinach-Stuffed Chicken 88

Strawberry Crepes 91

Conclusion 94

About the Author 95

Author's Afterthoughts 96

Introduction

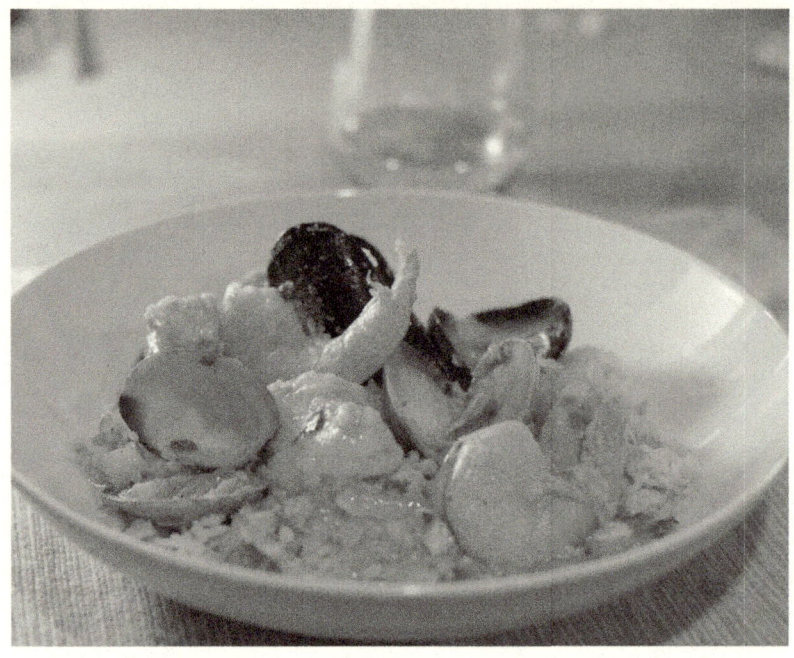

What is the HCG Diet? It is a diet which combines HCG injections and low-calorie eating. In recent times this diet has helped millions of people to achieve and maintain their ideal weight and keep healthy.

HCG (known as Human Chorionic Gonadotropin), a hormone that naturally occurs in the body. During a woman's pregnancy, this hormone is released by the placenta. Researches have shown that HCG injections combined with low-calorie diets can help individuals loose approximately two pounds daily if done properly. This combination can also help individuals to stay healthy and maintain a proper weight for the rest of their lives.

In this book, the recipes are meant to be accompanied by HCG injections daily and are geared for optimal success in weight loss. These recipes can assist you in losing weight even if you are not following the HCG diet properly and basically needs only a collection of low-calorie meal options. Since you are in it to win it, let's get started without any further ado.

Chocolate Mousse

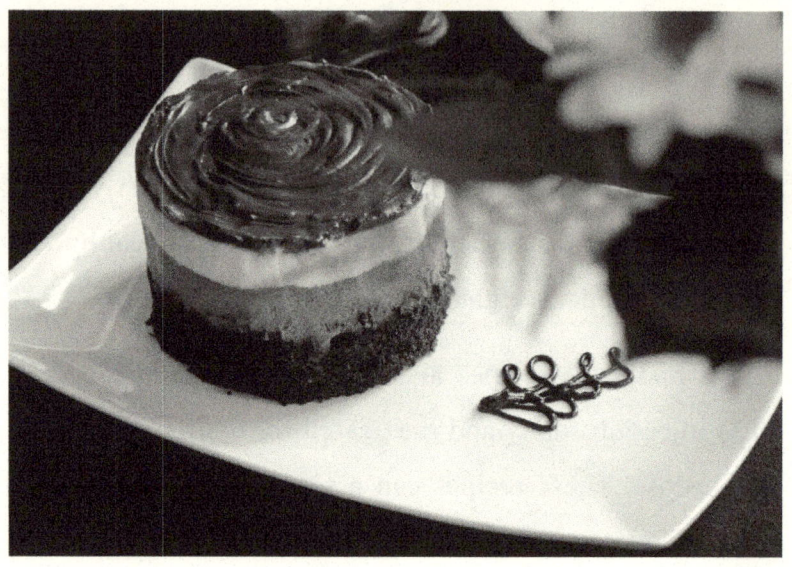

This delicious Chocolate Mousse is very versatile and nutritious

Time: 5 minutes + 1 hour chill time

Serves: 1

Ingredients:

- 1 tablespoon milk
- 1 tablespoon cocoa powder
- 0.5 cup low-fat or fat-free cottage cheese
- 1 teaspoon vanilla
- 1 tablespoons sugar substitute

Directions:

1. In a blender on low setting blend the cottage cheese until the cheese curds and become smooth.

2. Remove the cottage cheese from the blender and transfer to a mixing bowl.

3. To the blended cottage cheese, add the milk, cocoa powder, vanilla, and sugar substitute.

4. Use a spoon to mix thoroughly until ingredients are totally combined.

5. Chill in the refrigerator for 1 hour before serving.

6. Can be kept in an air-tight container in your refrigerator for approximately 5 days.

Asian Noodle Soup

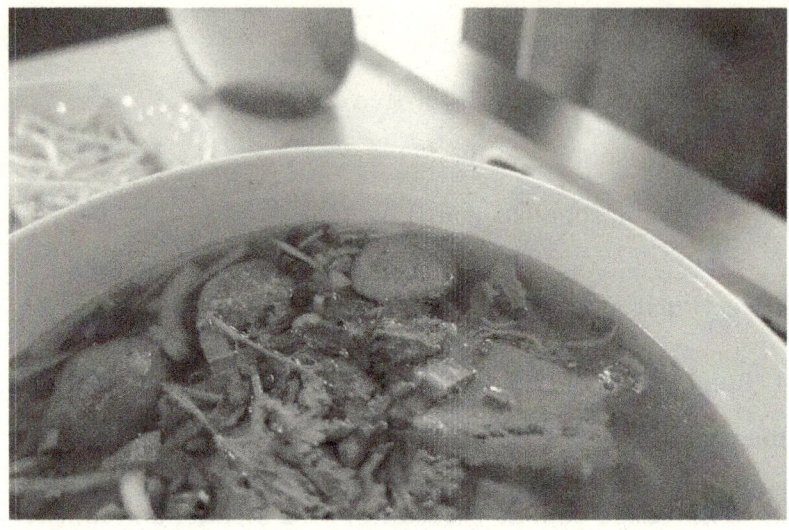

A great Asian Noodle Soup, very quick and easy to make.

Time: 31 minutes

Serves: 1

Ingredients:

- 1 tablespoon chopped cilantro
- 3 chopped green onions
- 0.75 cup chopped green cabbage
- 2 cups beef broth (make sure to choose a low sodium option)
- 30.5 ounces thinly sliced beef
- 0.25 teaspoon pepper
- 0.25 teaspoon salt
- 1 bay leaf
- 0.25 teaspoon ginger
- 0.5 teaspoon minced garlic
- 0.125 tablespoon tamari

Directions:

1. Begin by preparing the vegetables by washing the cabbage, cilantro, and green onions thoroughly.

2. On a large cutting board, remove a section of cabbage leaves from the cabbage head and chop the cabbage leaves until you have obtained 0.75 cup of chopped cabbage. Set it aside for later.

3. After washing the cilantro, select a few stems and finely chop them with a sharp knife. Set it aside for later.

4. Repeat the same process with the green onions, making sure they are also finely chopped. Set them aside.

5. In the sauce pan, pour the beef broth. Then add the onions, half of the cilantro, pepper, salt, bay leaf, ginger, garlic, and tamari.

6. Bring the entire broth mixture to a boil.

7. Once the beef broth is boiling, add the thinly sliced beef and the cabbage. Lower the burner's heat. Then cook the mixture for another 15-25 minutes, making sure the cabbage appears soft before you turn the burner off.

8. Soup should be served hot using the remaining chopped cilantro to garnish.

Basic Egg Omelet

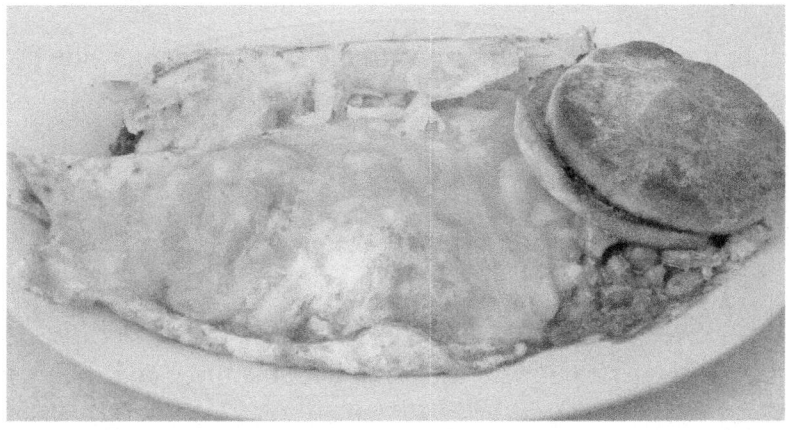

Master omelet making with this simple recipe then add the filling of your choice.

Time: 7 minutes

Serves: 1

Ingredients:

- 4 large eggs
- 1 tablespoon milk
- 0.5 teaspoon salt
- 0.5 teaspoon pepper
- 0.25 teaspoon parsley

Directions:

1. Over medium heat, heat a small frying pan.

2. In the small bowl crack one of the eggs and set it aside for later.

3. In the other small bowl, crack the remaining 3 eggs. With either a slotted spoon or another appropriate tool, take out the 3 yolks and discard them.

4. Add the first egg into the bowl with the three egg whites.

5. Add 1 tablespoon milk, salt, and pepper to the eggs. Whisk the eggs and spices rapidly. Ensure the egg mixture is frothy before moving on.

6. Add the egg mixture into a frying pan. Then cook for about 2 min. Wait for the edges of omelet begin to turn light brown before moving onto the next step.

7. After the omelet has begun to brown, using a spatula carefully flip half the omelet over on its other half. Give an additional 2 minutes for both sides.

8. Remove the frying pan from the heat and transfer the omelet to a plate. Garnish with the parsley and serve hot.

Cucumber Slices

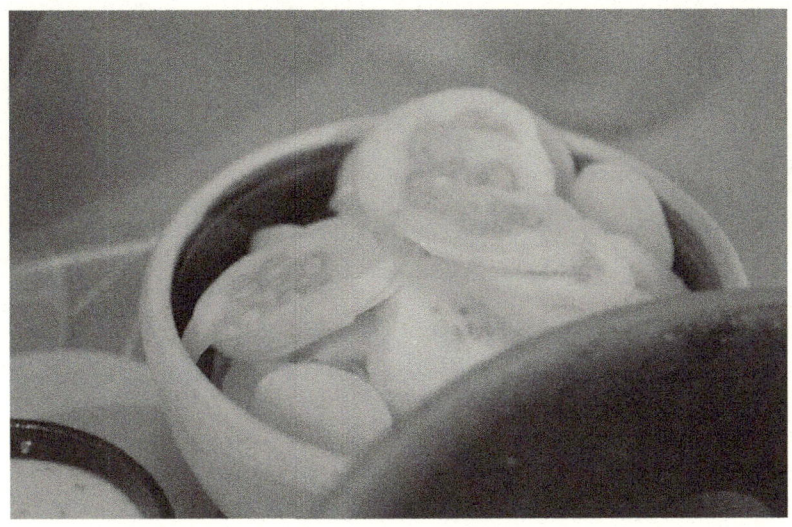

Refreshing Cucumber slices. Perfect topping for lettuce wraps, salads and meat dishes.

Time: 10 minutes

Serves: 1

Ingredients:

- 1 large cucumber
- 0.5 lemon
- 0.5 teaspoon salt
- 0.5 teaspoon pepper
- 0.125 teaspoon cumin

Directions:

1. Begin by preparing the cucumber by washing it thoroughly. You can also remove the peel of the cucumber if desired.

2. Cut the cucumber into small slices on a cutting board. Make sure that your slices are no thicker than 0.5 centimeters thick.

3. Once cut, place the cucumber slices into a zip-seal bag and set it aside for later.

4. Take half a lemon and using a lemon juicer or another appropriate tool, juice the lemon until you have obtained at least 1 tablespoon of lemon juice.

5. Add the lemon juice to the zip-seal bag along with the salt, pepper, and cumin.

6. Now seal the bag, shaking vigorously and ensuring that each cucumber slice is well coated with lemon juice and spices.

7. Open the bag and eat straight from the bag or transfer to a bowl and serve over a bed of chopped lettuce.

Classic Chicken Noodle Soup

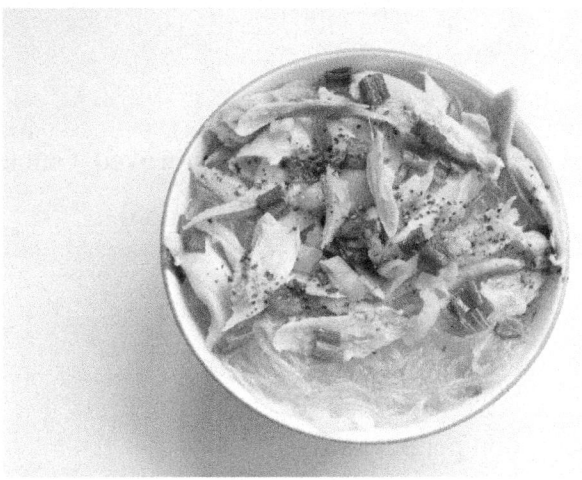

This is an all-time favorite Winter soup made with simple ingredients.

Time: 51 minutes

Serves: 1

Ingredients:

- 30.5 ounces of chicken breast
- 2 celery stalks
- 0.5 small onion
- 2 cups filtered water or HCG Approved Chicken Stock (recipe found in the Sauce section)
- 1 teaspoon oregano
- 1 teaspoon basil
- 0.5 teaspoon minced garlic
- 0.25 teaspoon pepper
- 10.25 teaspoon salt.

Directions:

1. On one of the cutting boards, place the 30.5 ounces of chicken breast and cut into 1-inch cubes. Be sure to remove any extra fat you see from the chicken.

2. Once the chicken is cut, pour the 2 cups of water in the small sauce pan and add the chicken.

3. Bring the water and chicken to a boil. After they are boiling, lower the burner's heat. Next, cover the sauce pan. Continue to boil for another 15 minutes, ensuring that the chicken is thoroughly cooked.

4. While the chicken is cooking, prepare the onion and celery by washing them well in cold water. Make sure to remove the onion skin before washing it.

5. Then take the other cutting board and knife and chop the celery stalks into small piece. Set it aside for later.

6. Take the onion and cut it in half. Take one half and chop it into small pieces. Set it aside for later.

7. Once the chicken has been cooked, take it out of the sauce pan and place it in a bowl.

8. To the remaining water, add the chopped vegetables, oregano, basil, pepper and salt.

9. Cover the spices and vegetables. Then bring it to a boil.

10. Once boiling, lower the burner's heat. Continue cooking the vegetables for another 20-30 minutes or until they appear soft.

11. Add the chicken back in the sauce pan. Cook it continually for another 5 minutes covered.

12. Serve the soup hot and enjoy.

Baked Apple Slices

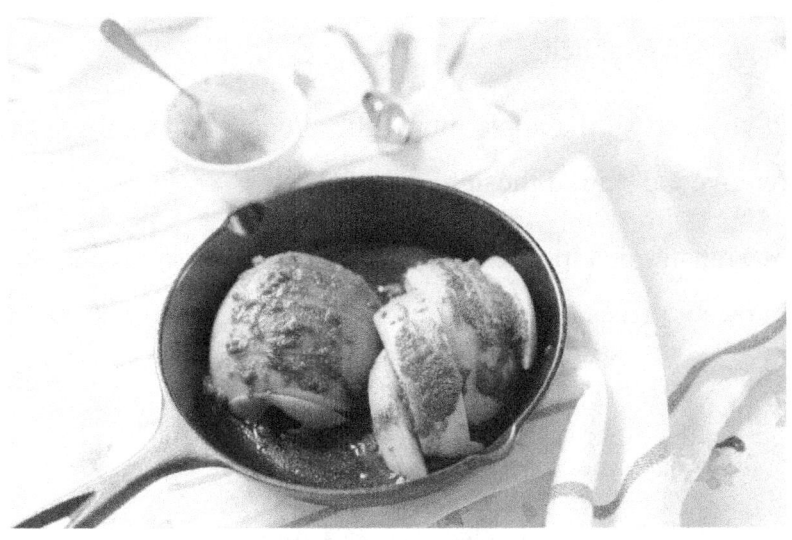

A very delicious way to enjoy your apples.

Time: 25 minutes

Serves: 1

Ingredients:

- 1 large apple
- 0.25 cup of filtered water
- 0.25 teaspoon cinnamon
- 0.5 teaspoon sugar substitute

Directions:

1. Put the conventional oven in a preheating setting for 350 degrees Fahrenheit.

2. Next, wash the apple thoroughly in cool water. You can remove the skin of the apple if you wish.

3. Transfer the apple to the cutting board and cut the apple into four pieces lengthwise.

4. Remove the apple's core and toss.

5. Take each piece of apple and cut into smaller slices.

6. Put the apple slices into a small dish that is oven-safe.

7. In another small bowl, join the spices together including the cinnamon, sugar substitute and filtered water.

8. Once mixed, pour the mixture over the top of the apples.

9. Place the apple slices in the conventional oven. Then bake the apple slices for approximately 15 minutes. You will want to make sure the apples are soft before taking them out of the oven.

10. Take out the baking dish and serve hot.

Chicken Curry Soup

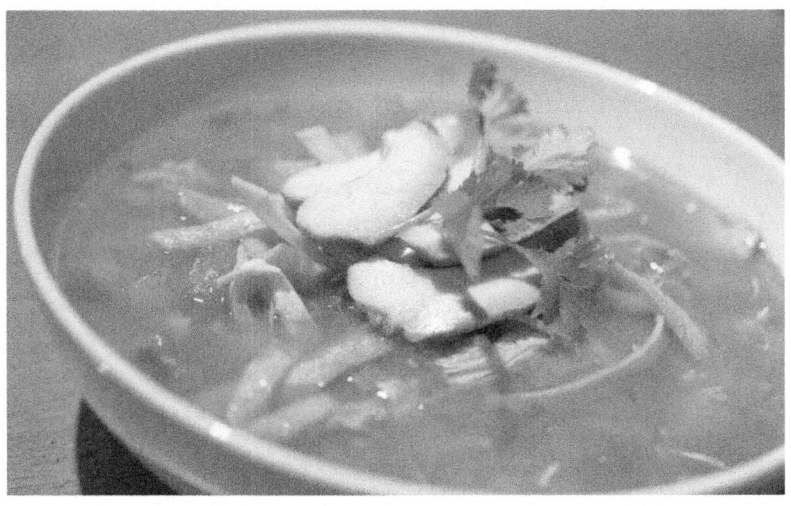

This is an amazing, healing one pot Chicken Curry Soup.

Time: 26 minutes

Serves: 1

Ingredients:

- 2 cups filtered water or HCG Approved Chicken Stock
- 30.5 ounces of chicken breast
- 1 small onion
- 1 garlic clove
- 0.25 teaspoon cinnamon
- 0.125 teaspoon ginger
- 0.125 teaspoon nutmeg
- 0.5 teaspoon curry powder

Directions:

1. On one of the cutting boards, place the 30.5 ounces of chicken breast and cut into 1-inch cubes. Be sure to remove any extra fat you see from the chicken.

2. Once the chicken is cut, pour the 2 cups of water in the small sauce pan and add the chicken.

3. Boil the water and chicken. When they are boiling, lower the burner's heat. Cover the sauce pan. Then, continue to boil for another 15 minutes. Make sure the chicken is thoroughly cooked before continuing to the next step.

4. During the cooking of the chicken, remove the skin of the onion and wash well with cold water.

5. Using the other cutting board and knife, chop the onion in to small pieces and Set it aside for later.

6. Using a sharp knife mince the garlic and set it aside as well.

7. Remove the chicken once it is cooked and set it aside.

8. Next, put the onions in the water as well as the garlic, curry powder, cinnamon, ginger, and nutmeg.

9. Wait for it to reach a boiling temperature and cover the onions in the water, cooking for approximately 5 minutes. Make sure the onions are soft before moving to the next step.

10. Add the chicken back to the water. Cover the sauce pan. Cook the chicken soup for 5 more minutes.

11. Take the soup off the burner and serve hot.

Savory Fish Stew

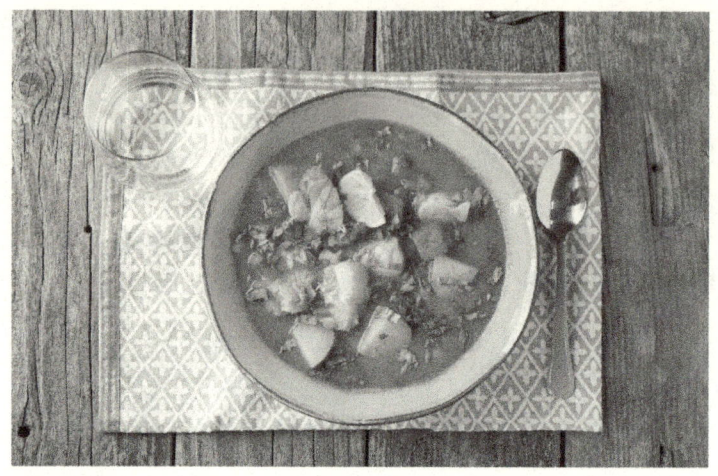

This Savory Fish Stew is flavorful, warming and light.

Time: 26 minutes

Serves: 1

Ingredients:

- 0.5 small onion
- 0.25 cup of filtered water or HCG Approved Chicken Stock (recipe found in the Sauce section)
- 1 garlic clove
- 30.5 ounces halibut
- 0.125 teaspoon thyme
- 0.125 teaspoon basil
- 0.25 teaspoon salt
- 0.125 teaspoon pepper
- 1 small tomato
- 1 bay leaf

Directions:

1. Begin by preparing the onion and garlic. Remove the skin of the onion and wash it well.

2. Chop the onion in half, cut one half into small pieces, and set it aside.

3. Take the clove of garlic, remove the casing, and cut it with a sharp knife until it is well minced. Set it aside as well.

4. Wash the small tomato thoroughly until clean. Use the sharp knife to cut the tomato into 1-inch cubes. Set it aside for later.

5. Add the 0.25 cup filtered water to a small sauce pan. Boil the water and continue boiling for 5 more minutes.

6. When the water is boiling, add the onion to the pot along with the minced garlic. Lower the burner's heat. Cook onions for roughly 7 minutes or until soft.

7. While the onion is cooking, take the halibut on the other cutting board, cut it into small, bite-sized pieces.

8. Once the onion appears soft, add the halibut chunks to the sauce pan and cook until the halibut appears flakey, approximately another 5 minutes.

9. Once the fish is cooked, add the tomato cubes, salt, thyme, pepper, basil, and bay leaf. Boil the entire mixture.

10. Once boiling, immediately lower the burner's heat. Then, you should simmer the soup for another 5-7 minutes. Do not take the soup off the burner until the flavors are well mixed.

11. Remove from the heat and serve hot.

Tomato Soup

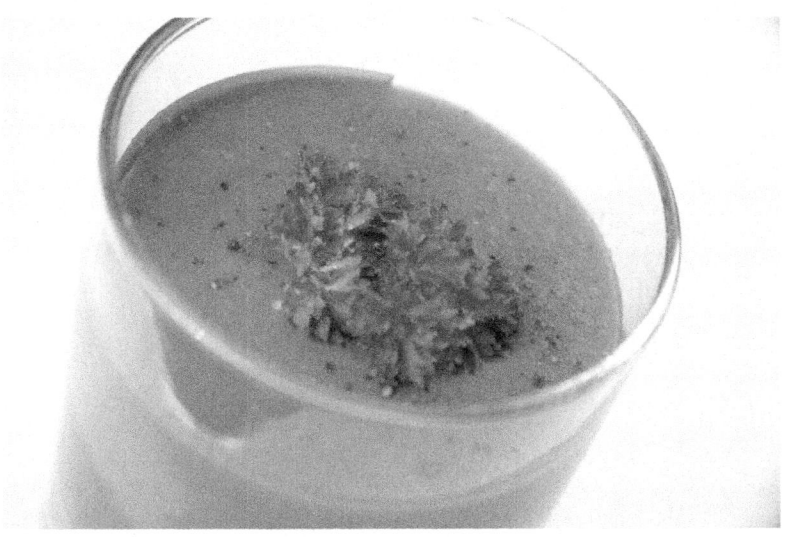

Need dinner in a hurry? This Tomato soup is the perfect choice, simple and delicious.

Time: 18 minutes

Serves: 1

Ingredients:

- 1 large tomato
- 10.5 ounces tomato paste
- 1 cup filtered water or HCG Approved Chicken Stock
- 1 small onion
- 1 tablespoon basil
- 1 garlic clove
- 0.25 teaspoon oregano
- 0.25 teaspoon of sugar substitute
- 0.125 teaspoon pepper
- 0.25 teaspoon salt

Directions:

1. Begin by preparing the vegetables. Wash the tomato and also, after the skin has been removed, wash the onion until both are clean.

2. On the cutting board, chop the tomato into small pieces. Add these pieces to the blender.

3. Chop the onion into small pieces and also add to the blender.

4. Remove the casing from the garlic clove and thoroughly mince it. Also, add it to the blender.

5. Measure out the basil, oregano, sugar substitute, pepper and salt. Add these spices to the blender.

6. Add the 10.5 ounces of tomato paste and the filtered water to the blender.

7. Blend the entire mixture on high for 1 minutes, or until the tomato and onion have been pulverized.

8. Transfer the mixture to a small sauce pan. Then bring the whole mixture to a boil. Continue to boil the soup for 7 more minutes.

9. Once the mixture is boiling, lower heat and cook it continually for another 5 minutes.

10. Remove from heat and serve hot.

Summertime Spinach Salad

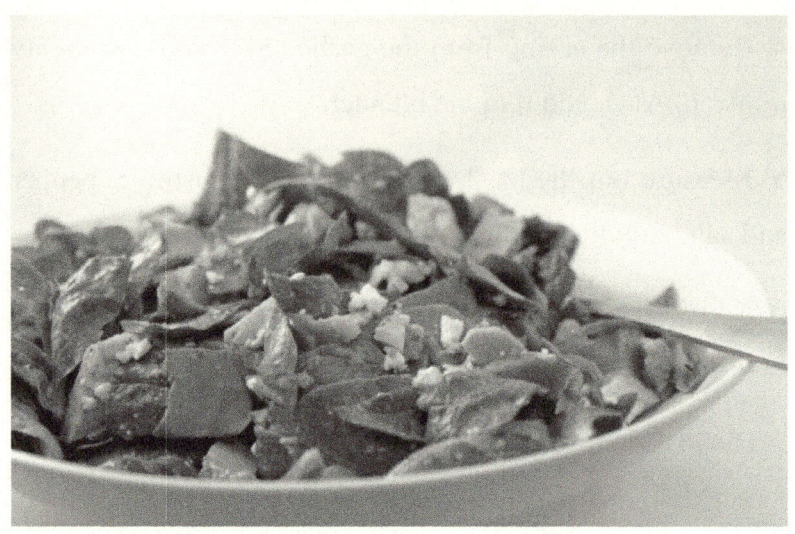

This salad is sweet, crunchy, quick and easy. Anti-oxidant rich and tasty.

Time: 10 minutes

Serves: 1

Ingredients:

- 1 cup spinach
- 5 strawberries
- 2 tablespoons dressing of your choice

Directions:

1. Begin by preparing the fruit and vegetables. Wash the 1 cup spinach and the 5 strawberries thoroughly.

2. Measure out the proper amount of spinach and transfer to the mixing bowl.

3. Next, take each strawberry and remove its stem. Then cut each strawberry into circular slices widthwise. Repeat with each strawberry. Transfer the sliced strawberries to the mixing bowl.

4. Measure out 2 tablespoons of the dressing of your choice. We recommend using either the Apple Cider Vinaigrette or the Citrus Dressing, the recipes for both of which can be found in the Sauces section.

5. Once all ingredients have been transferred to the mixing bowl, use the spatula and toss the spinach and strawberries until all vegetables and fruits are evenly coated with dressing.

6. Serve. Can also be stored in an air-tight container in the refrigerator for another 5 days

Low-Calorie Chili

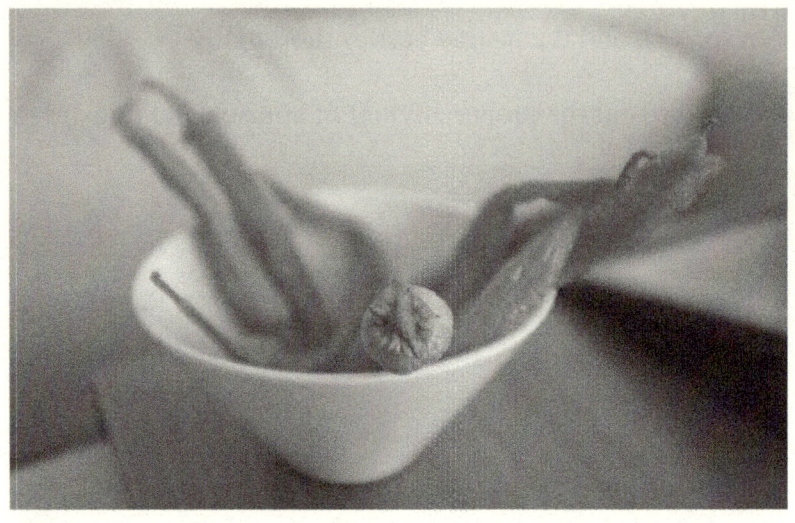

Low-Calorie Chili, a healthy choice for brunch or dinner.

Time: 20 minutes

Serves: 1

Ingredients:

- 0.125 teaspoon salt
- 0.125 teaspoon pepper
- 0.125 teaspoon cayenne pepper (or more if you like it extra spicy)
- 0.25 teaspoon oregano
- 0.25 teaspoon chili powder
- 10.5 teaspoon minced garlic
- 0.125 onion chopped
- 1 cup sliced tomato
- 0.5 cup filtered water or HCG Approved Chicken Stock
- 30.5 ounces ground beef make sure it is very lean

Directions:

1. Begin by preparing the vegetables and garlic.

2. Wash the tomato in cool water until clean. Using a cutting board and knife, slice the tomatoes into 0.25 square inch pieces or about that. Set it aside for later.

3. Be sure to remove the skin of the onion and cut out a portion of it about 0.125 of the entire onion. Then chop the onion and set it aside.

4. Remove the casing from the garlic and using the cutting board and knife, mince the garlic until you have about 10.5 teaspoons of it. Set it aside for later.

5. Once the vegetables have been prepared, remove any excess fat from the lean ground beef and brown it in a small frying pan.

6. When the beef has been cooked, add the chopped onions and minced garlic. Cook it continually until all the flavors are mixed together.

7. Stir in the chopped tomatoes and add the 0.5 cup filtered water.

8. Turn the heat of the burner down to simmer the beef and vegetables.

9. After about 2 minutes of simmering, add the spices one by one to the beef.

10. Continue simmering the mixture until most but not all of the water has evaporated.

11. After the beef and vegetables have simmered for about 10 minutes and most of the water is gone, it is ready to be served and can be served with additional onion as a garnish if desired.

HCG Approved Deviled Eggs

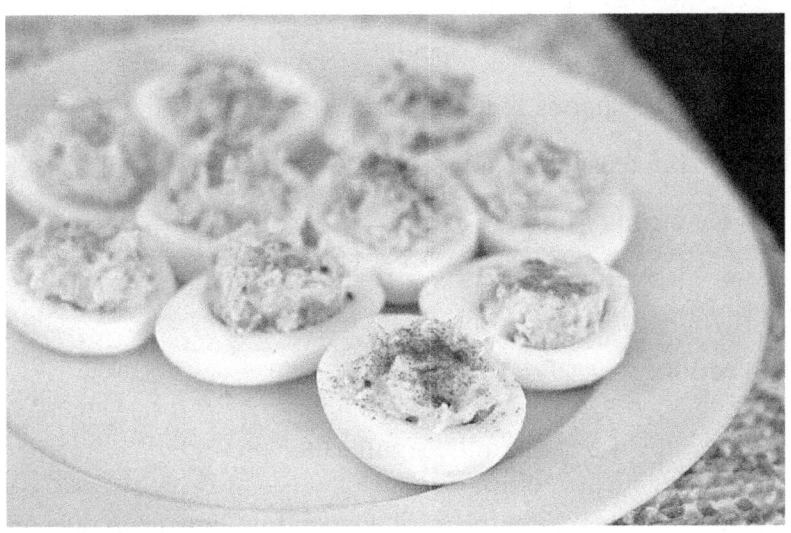

This deviled egg recipe is sure to let you lose weight. A great start to your day.

Time: 17 minutes

Serves: 2

Ingredients:

- 4 large eggs
- 0.25 teaspoon pepper
- 2 teaspoons Dijon mustard
- 0.5 teaspoon salt
- 2 cups filtered water
- 0.5 tablespoon milk

Directions:

1. Place the 4 eggs into the small sauce pan.

2. Pour the water over the eggs. Depending how deep the pan is you might need less water or more. You want the water to just cover the top of the eggs.

3. Place on the stove top and wait for it to reach a boiling temperature.

4. Lower the burner's heat and cover the pot. Then cook continually for another 12 minutes.

5. While the eggs are cooking, combine in a small-sized bowl the following ingredients Dijon mustard, pepper, milk, and salt.

6. Whisk together everything well and set it aside for later.

7. When the eggs are finished cooking, remove from heat and pour out the water.

8. Run cold water over the eggs for another minute.

9. Crack and peel the eggs.

10. Slice eggs in half and remove their yolks. Transfer the yolks to the bowl with the spices.

11. Using a fork, smash the cooked egg yolks into the spices. Whisk everything together until the egg yolks have been well combined with the spices.

12. Lay the empty egg white halves on a plate with scooped out part facing up. Scoop 1 tablespoon of egg yolk and spice mixture and place it in the empty egg whites. Repeat until all the egg white halves have been filled.

13. Eat immediately or you can keep these in the refrigerator for up to 3 days in an airtight container.

Tokyo Cucumber Salad

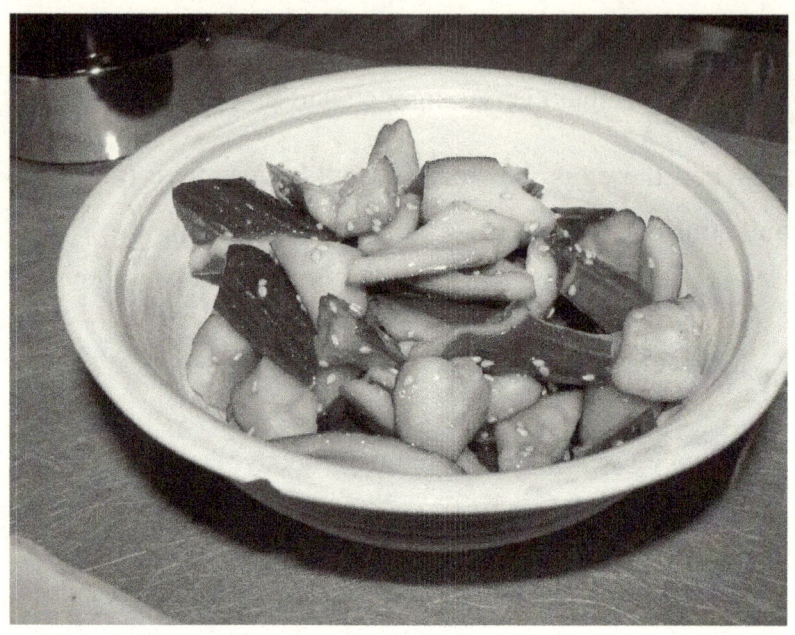

This is an easy salad enriched with vinegar and cucumber. Very light and delicious.

Time: 10 minutes

Serves: 1

Ingredients:

- 1 medium cucumber
- 1 garlic clove
- 0.25 teaspoon pepper
- 0.25 teaspoon salt
- 0.25 cup rice vinegar
- 1 teaspoon sugar substitute
- 10.5 teaspoon dried pepper flakes

Directions:

1. Begin by preparing the cucumber. Wash the cucumber thoroughly. You can also peel the cucumber if you do not like to eat the peel. Transfer the cucumber to the cutting board and chop the cucumber into slices no more than 1 centimeter thick.

2. Once you have chopped the entire cucumber into slices, cut each slice into smaller cubes, about 0.25 square centimeters. You want the cucumber to be finely chopped.

3. Move the chopped cucumber to a mixing bowl then set it aside.

4. Remove husk of the garlic clove and mince the garlic well. Place the minced garlic into the small bowl.

5. Add some rice vinegar to the garlic. Stir the whole mixture around with the spatula.

6. Then measure out the pepper, salt, dried pepper flakes, and sugar substitute. Add these spices to the bowl that contains the rice vinegar.

7. Mix the rice vinegar along with the spices together until everything is well combined.

8. Transfer the vinegar dressing to the mixing bowl.

9. Using the spatula, mix together the vegetables and dressing until everything is evenly coated with the dressing.

10. Serve immediately. You can also store the salad in an airtight container in the refrigerator for another 5 days.

Taco Salad

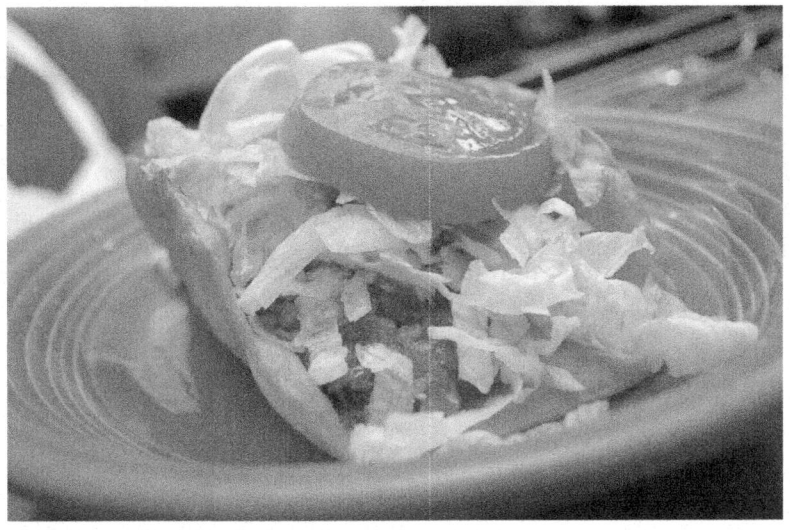

The whole family will love this healthy Taco Salad.

Time: 16 minutes

Serves: 1

Ingredients:

- 30.5 ounces lean ground beef
- 1 garlic clove
- 1 small tomato
- 0.5 teaspoon oregano
- 2 cups lettuce
- 1 teaspoon cumin
- 1 tablespoon chili powder
- 0.5 teaspoon salt

Directions:

1. Add the ground beef to a medium frying pan. Be sure to remove any extra fat you see before cooking.

2. Brown the beef, about 7 minutes, until it is cooked thoroughly.

3. While the meat is cooking, remove the husk from the garlic clove and mince it well. Set it aside for later.

4. When the meat has completed cooking remove it from the heat and add the minced garlic, chili powder, cumin, oregano, and salt. Using a spatula, stir the spices into the meat until everything is well combined. Set it aside.

5. Wash the lettuce and tomato. Remove the white part of the lettuce if you desire. Cut the lettuce into strips and transfer to the mixing bowl.

6. Remove the stem from the tomato and cut the entire tomato into 1-inch cubes. Transfer to the mixing bowl.

7. Add the spiced meat to the mixing bowl and with the spatula stir everything together until well combined.

8. Serve hot and eat immediately.

Grilled Chicken Salad

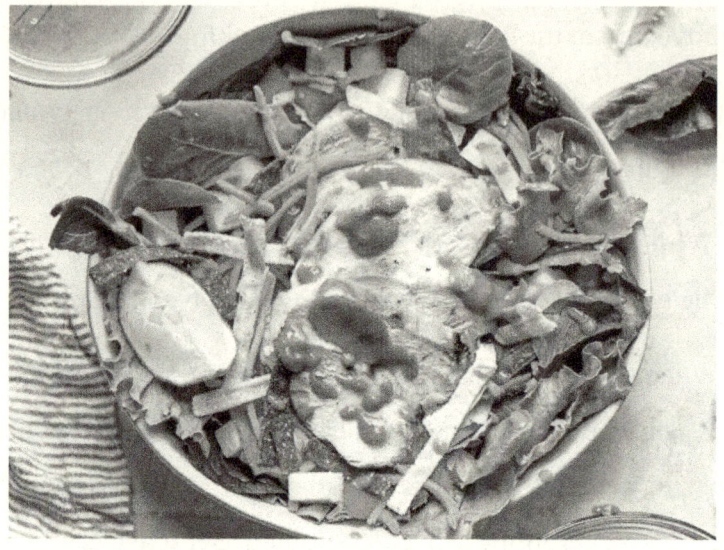

No fancy restaurant can beat this salad. Bursting with flavor and taste as good as it looks.

Time: 20 minutes

Serves: 1

Ingredients:

- 30.5 ounces chicken breast
- 0.25 teaspoon salt
- 0.25 teaspoon pepper
- 1 small apple
- 3 celery stalks
- 0.5 lemon
- 0.25 teaspoon cinnamon
- 0.25 teaspoon nutmeg
- 0.25 teaspoon sugar substitute

Directions:

1. Combine the pepper and salt together in a small bowl to make a rub for the chicken. Add the pepper and salt together with the chicken breasts and spread until the chicken breast is fully covered.

2. Then, put the chicken breast into a small frying pan. Next, grill the chicken until thoroughly cooked. You can grill it for about 15 minutes. Remove the chicken from burner's heat and transfer to the cutting board.

3. Cut the grilled chicken into approximate cubes and place in the mixing bowl.

4. Wash the apple and celery thoroughly. You can remove the apple peel if you wish. Transfer the apple and celery to the cutting board and cut the apple into approximate cubes. You can remove the stem and the core of the apple at this time. Next, transfer the apple slices to the bowl you will use for mixing.

5. Cut the celery into slices, ensure that no slice is wider than 0.5 centimeters. Transfer the celery slices to the mixing bowl.

6. Wash the lemon and cut in half. Using a lemon juicer or another appropriate tool, juice the lemon until you have about 2 tablespoons worth of juice. place in a separate small bowl.

7. In this bowl, combine the cinnamon, nutmeg, and sugar substitute together with the lemon juice. Whisk together until all the spices are will combined with the lemon juice.

8. Drizzle the lemon juice and spices over the chicken, apple, and celery.

9. Using the spatula, mix together the vegetables, fruit, chicken, and dressing until everything is evenly coated with the dressing.

10. Serve immediately or you can store the salad in the refrigerator in an air-tight container for another 5 days.

Fried Chicken Tenders

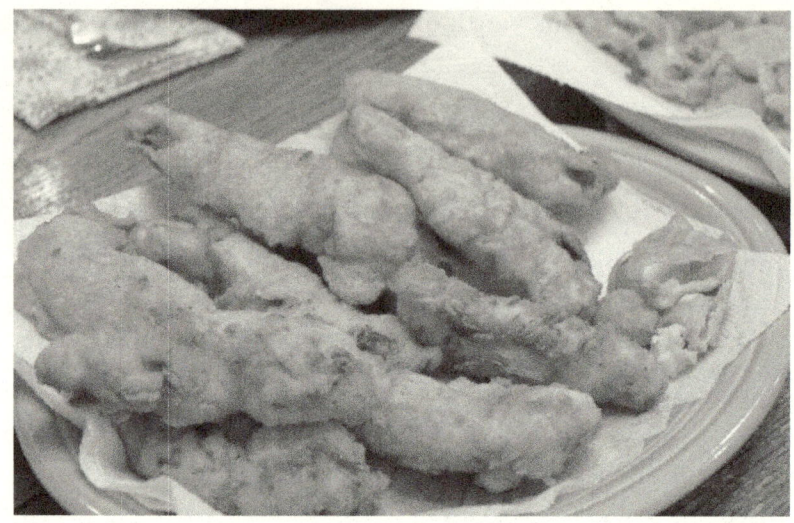

You will definitely love this. Really crispy, juicy and tasty.

Time: 36 minutes

Serves: 1

Ingredients:

- 30.5 ounces chicken breast
- 1 tablespoon milk
- 0.25 teaspoon salt
- 0.125 teaspoon pepper
- 0.125 teaspoon oregano
- 0.125 teaspoon red pepper flakes
- 1 grissini breadstick

Directions:

1. Preheat a conventional oven to 350 degrees Fahrenheit.

2. Take the chicken breast and cut it into 3 separate pieces. Make sure to remove any visible fat from the chicken at this time. Set it aside.

3. In a small mixing bowl, join the milk with the salt, pepper, oregano, and red pepper flakes. Set it aside.

4. In a zip-seal bag place the grissini breadstick.

5. Using the bottom of a glass cup crush the grissini breadstick until it is nothing but crumbs. Set it aside for later.

6. Take one of the chicken breast pieces and dip it in the milk and spices. Then place it in the zip-seal bag and shake for 15 seconds. Transfer the chicken from the bag to an oven-safe baking dish.

7. Repeat this process for each piece of chicken, making sure to coat them all evenly with spices and the bread crumbs.

8. Place the oven-safe baking dish into the conventional oven. Bake the chicken for 15 minutes.

9. After 15 minutes, rotate the chicken onto its back side and bake for an additional 10 minutes.

10. Then for the remaining few minutes, turn on the oven's broiler setting and broil for about 2 minutes.

11. Serve immediately.

Shredded Barbecue Chicken Salad

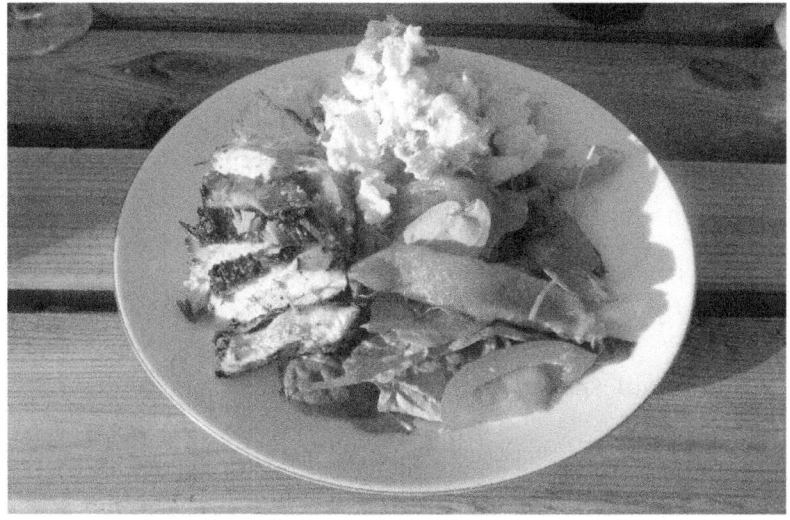

This chicken salad is darn delicious, flavorful and healthy!

Time: 21 minutes

Serves: 1

Ingredients:

- 1 cup water
- 30.5 ounces chicken breast
- 2 tablespoons vinegar
- 2 cups lettuce
- 0.5 tablespoon Dijon mustard
- 1 tablespoon sugar
- 1 teaspoon salt
- 1 tablespoon tomato paste
- 1 teaspoon pepper
- 1 teaspoon hot sauce

Directions:

1. Add the 1 cup water to the sauce pan and add the chicken. Allow the chicken to boil, then cover. Next, lower the burner's heat and continue cooking for another 15 minutes. Ensure the chicken is thoroughly cooked before moving on to the next step.

2. Once the chicken has been cooked, remove the chicken from the water (now chicken stock). Transfer the cooked chicken to the cutting board.

3. Using the two forks, shred the chicken thoroughly, transfer to the bowl you will use for mixing, then set it aside.

4. In a different bowl, combine the vinegar, salt, sugar, pepper, tomato paste, Dijon mustard, and hot sauce. Whisk together well making sure that everything is combined.

5. Transfer the dressing to the mixing bowl and pour it over the shredded chicken.

6. Using the spatula, coat the shredded chicken with the dressing until evenly covered.

7. Wash the lettuce and chop into strips. You can remove the white parts of the lettuce if you want to.

8. Add the lettuce to the bowl you are using for mixing. Combine the lettuce with the chicken using tossing motions.

9. Serve immediately or you can keep the salad in an air-tight container in a refrigerator for another 5 days.

Hard-Boiled Egg Salad

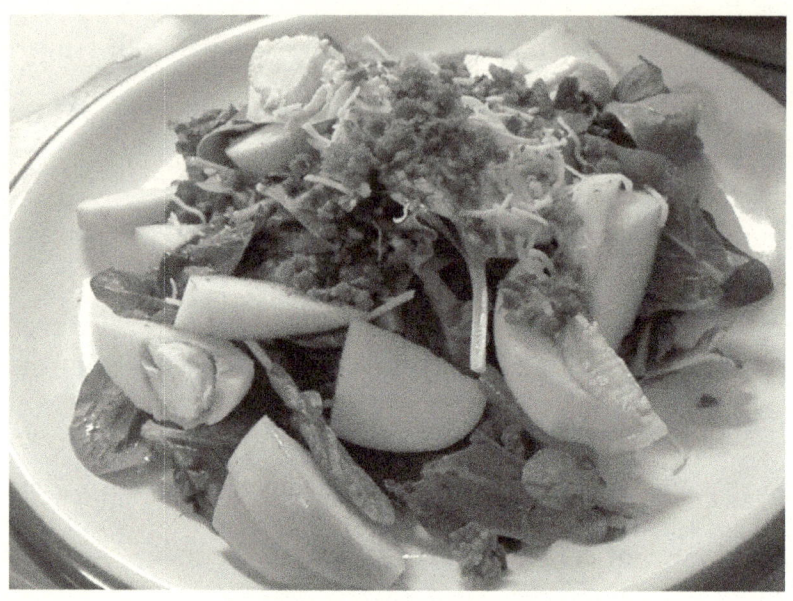

One of the best Egg Salad ever. Very simple and nutritious.

Time: 17 minutes

Serves: 1

Ingredients:

- 4 large eggs
- 1 cup of lettuce
- 1 tablespoon milk
- 0.5 teaspoon salt
- 0.25 teaspoon pepper
- 1 teaspoon Dijon mustard

Directions:

1. Place the 4 eggs into the small sauce pan.

2. Poor the water over the eggs. You might need more water or less depending on the depth of the pan. You want the water to just cover the top of the eggs.

3. Place on the stove top and wait for it to reach a boiling temperature.

4. Lower the burner's heat and cover the pot. Then cook continually for another 12 minutes.

5. While the eggs are cooking, wash the lettuce and move it to the surface you will use for cutting. Using the sharp life, cut the lettuce in to pieces, arrange it on a plate, and set it aside for later.

6. In a small bowl, join the following together: 1 tablespoon milk, salt, pepper, and Dijon mustard. Whisk together until everything is well combined.

7. When the eggs are finished cooking, remove from heat and pour out the water.

8. Run cold water over the eggs for another minute.

9. Crack and peel the eggs.

10. Slice eggs in half and remove 3 of the yolks. Discard them.

11. Place the eggs in the bowl with the combine spices, and using a fork, mash everything together making sure you combine all the ingredients together.

12. Place the mashed egg mixture over the bed of lettuce and serve immediately.

Beef-Stuffed Cabbage Rolls

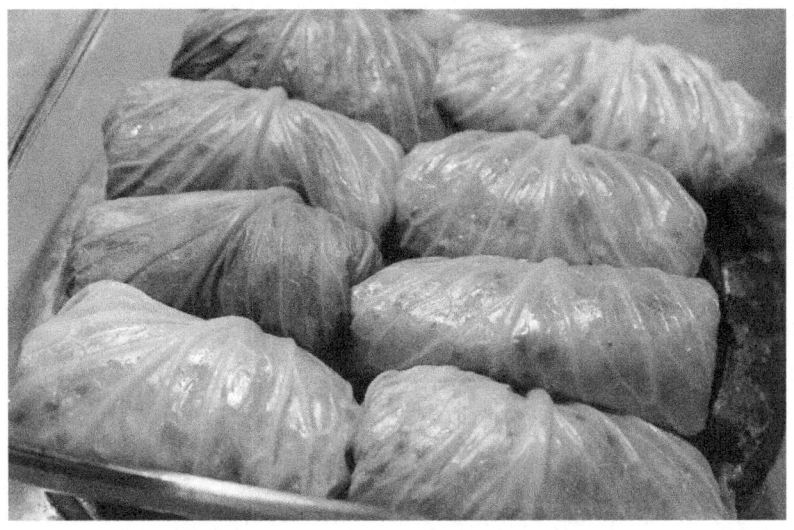

Delicious comfort food for a great family dinner.

Time: 25 minutes

Serves: 1

Ingredients:

- 30.5 ounces lean ground beef
- 3 large cabbage leaves
- 0.125 onion
- 1 garlic clove
- 0.5 teaspoon sugar substitute
- 0.25 teaspoon ginger

Directions:

1. Begin by preparing the vegetables. Wash the cabbage leaves thoroughly and set into a vegetable steamer. Steam for about 5 minutes. Before removing the cabbage leaves, you will want them to appear slightly limp so they will be easier to roll up. Take the leaves out of the pot and cut each one in half.

2. Additionally, remove the skin from the onion and wash.

3. Transfer the onion to the cutting board and slice of a piece about 0.125 of the entire onion. Chop this small section into more small pieces and place into the frying pan.

4. Take the husk from off the garlic clove and mince well. Also, add the minced garlic.

5. Join the ground beef with the other ingredients in the frying pan, making sure to remove any extra fat you see before cooking.

6. Using the spatula, push the ground beef into the chopped onions and minced garlic. Cook until beef is well cooked, about 10 minutes.

7. Once beef is cooked, add the 0.5 teaspoon sugar substitute and the 0.25 teaspoon garlic to the meet.

8. Remove the beef from the heat and using a tablespoon, add 20.5 tablespoons of the meat mixture to one of the cabbage leaf halves. Repeat this process until all the cabbage leaves are full.

9. Now you are going to roll the cabbage leaves. Take two opposite sides of the cabbage leaf and fold them in towards the middle of the leaf. Press down, and while holding these two sides down, take the other two opposite sides and fold them down and tuck one side in the other. Flip the cabbage roll over and place on a plate.

10. Serve these hot or cold.

Mongolian Beef Bowl

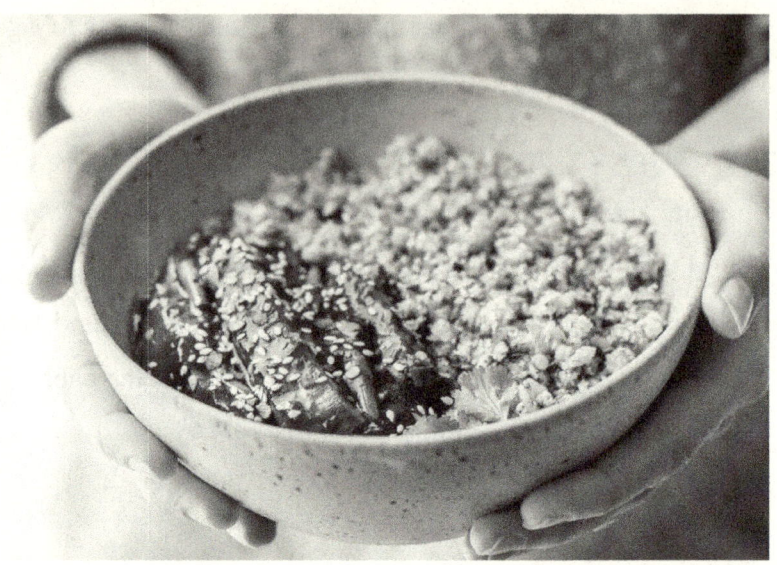

You can skip takeout and enjoy this tasty Mongolian Beef Bowl.

Time: 16 minutes

Serves: 1

Ingredients:

- 30.5 ounces of thinly sliced beef
- 0.125 head of cabbage
- 1 orange, for juicing
- 0.5 cup filtered water
- 1 lemon, for juicing
- 1 garlic clove
- 1 tablespoon apple cider vinegar
- 0.25 teaspoon chili powder
- 2 tablespoons tamari
- 0.25 teaspoon salt
- 0.125 teaspoon pepper

Directions:

1. Prepare the cabbage by washing it with cold water.

2. Transfer it to a cutting board and chop it into small slices. Set it aside for later.

3. Take half a lemon and using a lemon juicer or another appropriate tool, juice the lemon until you have collected 2 tablespoons worth of juice. Repeat the same process with the orange, collecting 2 tablespoons worth of orange juice. Set it aside for later.

4. Remove the husk of the garlic clove and mince the garlic well. Set it aside for later.

5. Pour both the lemon and orange juice into a small bowl. Combine with the fruit juices the apple cider vinegar, the water, and the tamari.

6. Mix in the salt, pepper, minced garlic, and chili powder. Whisk everything together making sure you combine all the ingredients well. Set it aside for later.

7. In the frying pan, place the slices of beef and cook on medium heat for 2 minutes.

8. Join the cabbage with the other ingredients and cook it continually for another 2 minutes.

9. Join the liquid to the ingredients and continue cooking for another 5 to 7 minutes. Make sure that the beef is has been well cooked and the cabbage appears soft before moving onto the next step.

10. Remove from heat and serve immediately.

Tilapia del Rio

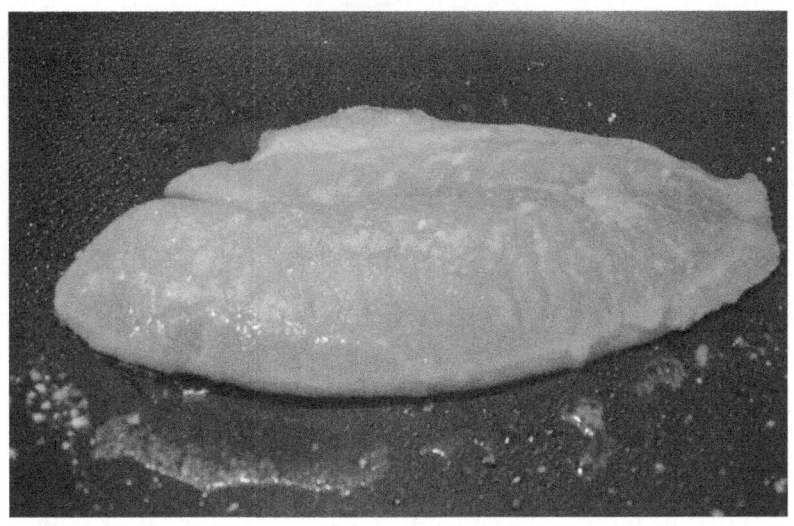

Fresh, flavorful and nutritious. Ready in a jiffy.

Time: 31 minutes

Serves: 1

Contains: 1 protein serving, 0.5 fruit serving

Ingredients:

- 30.5 ounces of tilapia fillet
- 0.5 lemon
- 1 teaspoon salt
- 0.5 teaspoon pepper
- 5 stems of cilantro

Directions:

1. Put the oven on a preheating setting to warm the oven up to 425 degrees Fahrenheit.

2. Wash the lemon and using the lemon zester or a cheese grater, zest the lemon into a small bowl.

3. In the same small bowl, combine the pepper and salt. Mix together until everything is well combined.

4. Take the cilantro stems and wash them thoroughly. Then chop them into small pieces. Set it aside for later.

5. On the cutting board, slice the lemon into thin slices, ensuring that they are no more than 0.5 centimeters thick.

6. Take the tilapia fillet and rub the salt, pepper, and lemon zest onto both sides of the fillet.

7. Lay the tilapia fillet onto a piece of aluminum foil that is twice as big as the fillet itself.

8. Next, lay lemon slices atop the fillet, layering them just slightly. Sprinkle the cilantro pieces over the top of the lemon.

9. Fold the tinfoil over the fillet and fold each side over itself to create a seal.

10. Place the tinfoil with the fillet inside an oven-safe baking dish.

11. Next, put the baking dish into the oven. Bake the fish for 20 to 25 minutes. Make sure the fish is cooked thoroughly before taking it out of the oven.

12. Serve immediately.

Applesauce

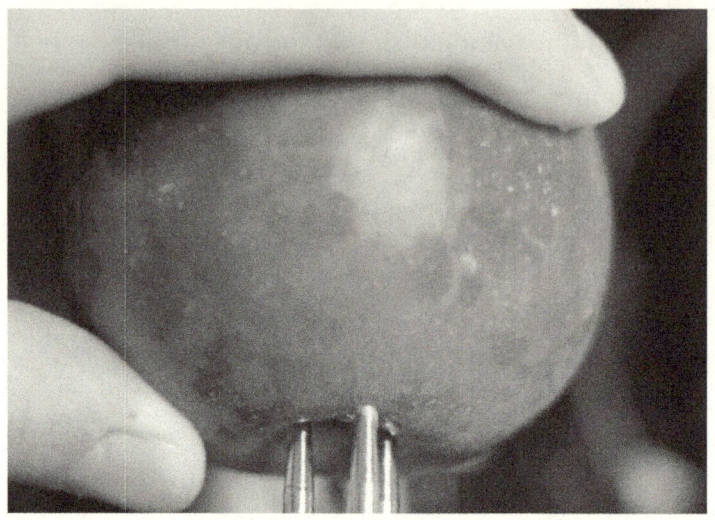

There is nothing better than rich homemade applesauce, made from freshly picked apples.

Time: 2 hours and 10 minutes

Serves: 1

Ingredients:

- 1 large apple
- 1 teaspoon sugar substitute
- 1 teaspoon cinnamon
- 3 tablespoons filtered water

Directions:

1. Begin by preparing the fruit by washing the apple thoroughly. You can remove the skin from the apple if you want.

2. Move the apple to the cutting board, and chop it into 0.25-inch cubes, removing the stem and core from the apple while doing so.

3. Place the apple chunks into the small sauce pan. Also add the water, cinnamon, and sugar substitute.

4. Cook the apple mixture on low for about 2 hours or until the apples are soft. It is wise to check the sauce pan about every 30 minutes to ensure that the apples are not overcooked.

5. Once the apples are soft and well-cooked, take the applesauce off of the hot burner.

6. Then take the potato masher or fork and smash the apples until they are the desired consistency. You can make the applesauce chunky or smoother depending on how long you mash the apples for.

7. You can serve this dish warm, or place in the refrigerator and serve cold.

Scrumptious Scrambled Eggs

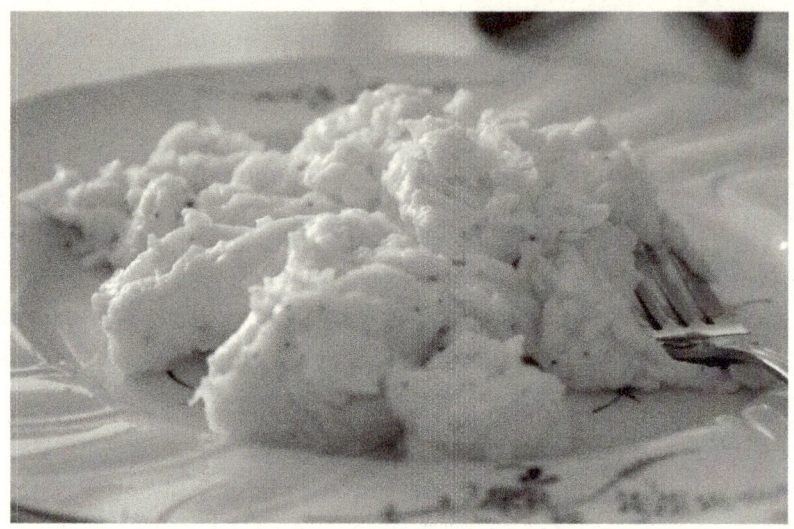

Scrumptious Scrambled Eggs, a delightful healthy breakfast.

Time: 12 minutes

Serves: 1

Ingredients:

- 0.5 small onion
- 0.5 cup spinach
- 4 large eggs
- 1 tablespoon milk
- 0.5 teaspoon salt
- 0.25 teaspoon pepper

Directions:

1. Prepare the vegetables by washing the spinach and setting aside.

2. Remove the skin from the onion and wash thoroughly. Transfer to the cutting board and chop the onion in half. Dice half the onion into small pieces and set it aside for later.

3. Over medium heat place a small frying pan.

4. In the small bowl crack one of the eggs and set it aside for later.

5. In the other small bowl, crack the remaining 3 eggs. With either a slotted spoon or another appropriate tool, take out the 3 yolks and discard them.

6. Add the first egg into the bowl with the three egg whites.

7. Add 1 tablespoon milk, salt, and pepper to the eggs. Whisk the eggs and spices rapidly. Ensure the egg mixture is frothy before moving on.

8. Add the egg mixture into a frying pan. Then join the eggs with the onions and spinach. Push the mixture around until everything is well combined. Let sit and cook for 2 minutes

9. Once again, push the mixture around using the spatula and let cook for another 2 minutes. Repeat this process until the eggs are thoroughly cooked, about 3 times.

10. Remove from heat and serve immediately.

Sloppy Joes

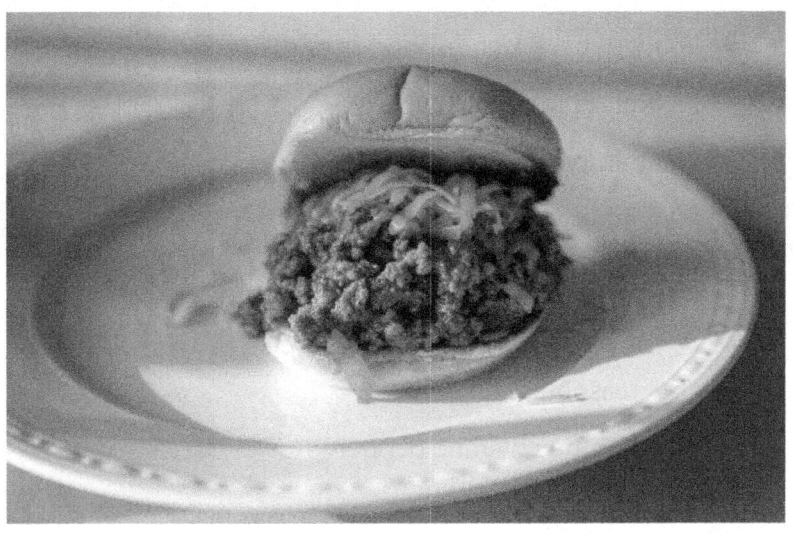

Step away from take-outs and give these homemade Sloppy Joes a try. You will totally enjoy!

Total: 16 minutes

Serves: 1

Ingredients:

- 3 lettuce leaves
- 30.5 ounces lean ground beef
- 3 ounces tomato paste
- 1 tablespoon Dijon mustard
- 0.5 onion
- 1 teaspoon salt
- 2 teaspoons sugar substitute
- 0.5 teaspoon pepper
- 1 teaspoon cayenne pepper

Directions:

1. Prepare the lettuce by selecting 3 leaves and washing them thoroughly. Set it aside for later.

2. Remove the skin from the onion and chop it well. Set it aside for later.

3. In a medium frying pan, begin to cook the ground beef. Be sure to remove any visible fat before cooking.

4. As the meat is cooking, add the tomato paste, salt, pepper, sugar substitute, Dijon mustard, cayenne pepper, and chopped onion.

5. Push around the meat and other ingredients, making sure to combine them well.

6. When the meat is cooked and the onions appear soft, remove from heat.

7. Fill each leaf of lettuce with about .3 of the meat mixture.

8. Serve hot and eat immediately.

Radish Chips

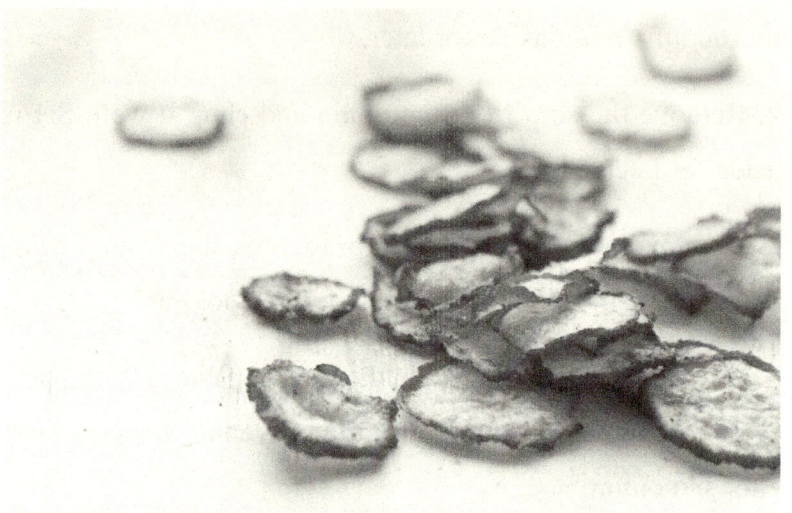

Crunchy low carb snack and a great side dish.

Time: 25 minutes

Serving: 1

Ingredients:

- 4 radishes
- 1 teaspoon salt
- 0.25 teaspoon pepper

Directions:

1. Put the conventional oven on a preheating setting for 375 degrees Fahrenheit.

2. Place parchment paper on a sheet used for baking and set it aside for later.

3. Begin by washing the radishes well in cold water.

4. Move to the cutting board and thinly slice each radish. Make sure that the width of each radish is no more than 0.25 centimeters. But the thinner the radish slices, the crispier the chips will come out.

5. Transfer the radish slice to a paper towel. On top of the radish slices lay another sheet of paper towel and press down, trying to remove any extra water from the radishes.

6. Lay the radish slices out on the baking sheet covered with parchment paper. Make sure that the slices don't overlap.

7. Sprinkle the radish slices with the measured-out pepper and salt.

8. Transfer the radish slices to a conventional oven and cook for 5 minutes.

9. Flip the radish slices over and continue cooking for another 10 minutes. You will want the edges of the radishes to be curling before you remove it from the oven.

10. After cooking, let the radish chips cool down some before eating them. Eat as a snack or side to a soup.

Dijon Mustard Chicken

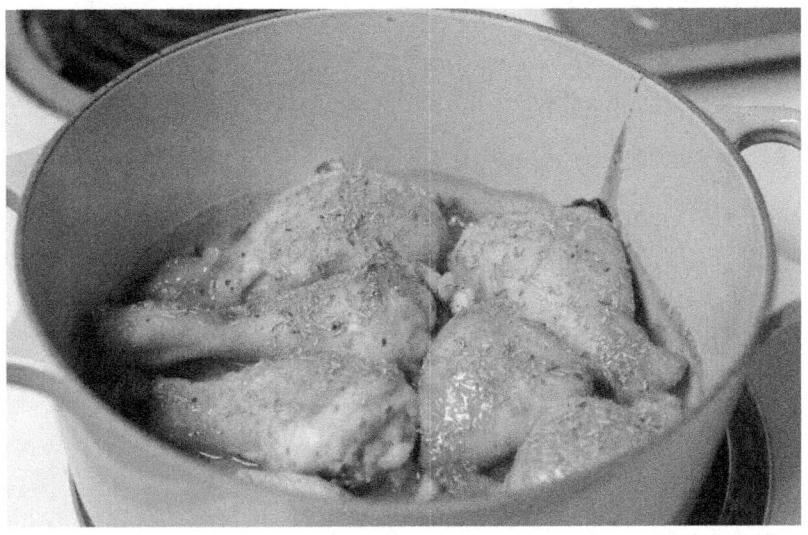

With just the right portion of zing and zest, this Dijon Mustard Chicken is just right for you.

Time: 30.5 hours and 10 minutes

Serves: 1

Ingredients:

- 30.5 ounces chicken breast
- 0.5 lemon
- 10.5 teaspoons lemon zest
- 0.25 teaspoon salt
- 1 garlic clove
- 2 tablespoons Dijon mustard
- 1 teaspoon rosemary
- 0.125 teaspoon pepper

Directions:

1. Begin by cutting a lemon in half and using a lemon juicer or another appropriate tool, juice the lemon, ensuring to collect at least 2 tablespoons worth of lemon juice.

2. Put the lemon juice in a bowl you will use for mixing. Set it aside for later.

3. Once the lemon is juiced, using a lemon zester, zest the lemon collection at least 10.5 teaspoons of lemon zest. Combine in the mixing bowl that contains the lemon juice.

4. Remove the garlic clove's husk and mince it well. Combine in the mixing bowl with the lemon juice as well.

5. Add the Dijon mustard and rosemary to the lemon juice. Whisk all together until the ingredients are thoroughly combined.

6. Place the chicken breast in a zip-seal bag. Pour the lemon juice mixture into the bag and seal it tight.

7. Place the bag with the chicken in the fridge and let marinate for at least 4 hours. The longer the chicken marinates, the more potent the flavors will be.

8. Once the chicken has thoroughly marinated, put the chicken in the oven-safe dish.

9. Bake the chicken for 10 minutes at 400 degrees Fahrenheit.

10. When the chicken is cooked, take it out and serve immediately.

Mexican Egg Omelet

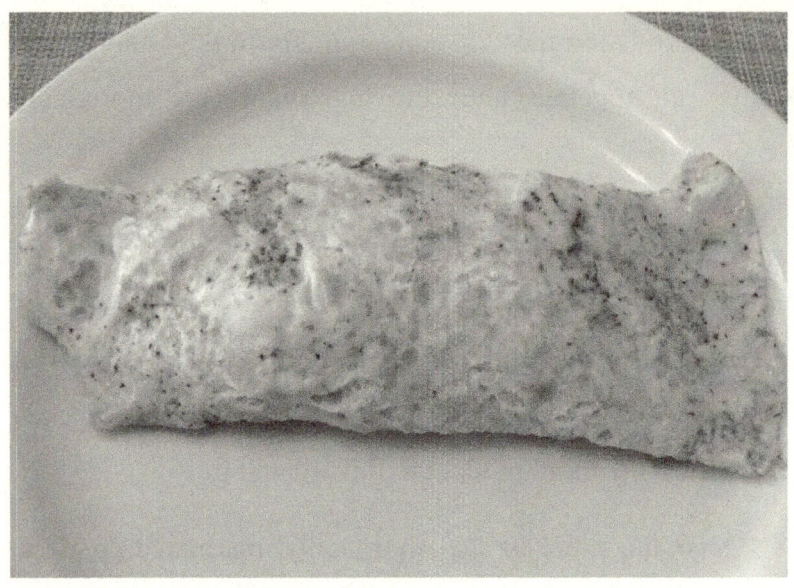

Incredibly delicious, stuffed with your favorite fresh ingredients.

Time: 15 minutes

Serves: 1

Ingredients:

- 4 large eggs
- 0.5 teaspoon salt
- 1 tablespoon milk
- 0.25 teaspoon pepper
- 1 small tomato
- 0.25 teaspoon chili powder
- 0.25 teaspoon oregano

Directions:

1. Prepare the tomato by washing it and cutting off its stem.

2. Transfer the tomato to a cutting board and cut it in to .5-inch square pieces. Set it aside for later.

3. In the small bowl crack one of the eggs and set it aside for later.

4. In the other small bowl, crack the remaining 3 eggs. With either a slotted spoon or another appropriate tool, take out the 3 yolks and discard them.

5. Add the first egg into the bowl with the three egg whites.

6. Add 1 tablespoon milk, salt, pepper, and chili powder to the eggs. Whisk the eggs. You will want the entire egg mixture to appear frothy.

7. Poor the egg mixture into the frying pan and cook for 2 minutes. You will know that the omelet is cooked when the edges begin to turn light brown.

8. Place the chopped tomatoes atop the omelet.

9. After the omelet has begun to brown, using a spatula carefully flip half the omelet over on its other half, covering the tomatoes. Cook for an additional 2 minutes on both sides.

10. Take away the frying pan from the burner's heat. Then, transfer the omelet to a plate. Garnish with the oregano and serve hot.

HCG Approved Crab Cakes

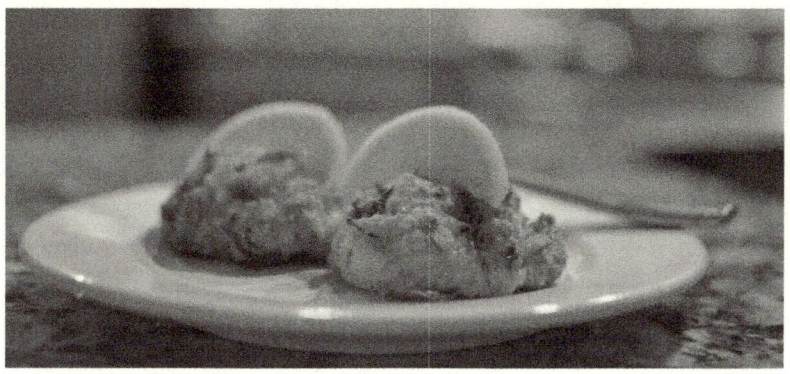

Special seafood appetizer. You can create this restaurant favorite from the comfort of your own kitchen.

Time: 21 minutes

Serves: 1

Ingredients:

- 1 garlic clove
- 1 lemon
- 1 grissini breadstick
- 10.5 teaspoon parsley flakes
- 0.5 teaspoon salt
- 0.25 teaspoon pepper
- 0.25 teaspoon red pepper flakes
- 30.5 ounces crab meat

Directions:

1. Preheat a conventional oven to 350 degrees Fahrenheit.

2. Remove the husk from the garlic, and mince thoroughly. Set into a medium bowl you will use for mixing and set it aside for later.

3. Wash the lemon before using a lemon zester or a cheese grater to collect 2 teaspoons lemon zest. Add to the small mixing bowl with the garlic.

4. With the remaining lemon, use a lemon juicer or another appropriate tool and collect 2 tablespoons worth of lemon juice into another small mixing bowl. Set it aside for later.

5. Place the grissini breadstick into a zip-seal bag. Smash the breadstick with the bottom of a glass cup until it is nothing but crumbs. Add the crumbs to the bowl in which you place the lemon juice.

6. In the same bowl, add the parsley flakes, salt, pepper, red pepper flakes, crab meat, and 1 tablespoon lemon juice. Mix everything together making sure you combine all the ingredients together thoroughly.

7. In an oven-safe baking dish, add the remaining lemon juice.

8. Break up the crab meat mixture into portions of equal sizes, about 4 portions. Place each portion into the baking dish.

9. Bake the cakes until they appear golden brown, roughly 15 minutes.

10. Remove and serve immediately.

Spinach-Stuffed Chicken

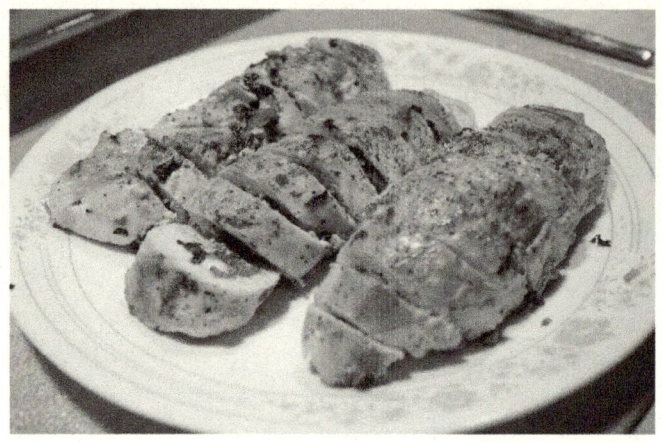

An exotic recipe with a rich, creamy, flavored spinach stuffing.

Time: 40 minutes

Serves: 1

Ingredients:

- 30.5 ounces chicken breast
- 1 garlic clove
- 0.5 teaspoon salt
- 0.25 teaspoon pepper
- 0.5 teaspoon rosemary
- 10-12 spinach leaves
- 1 cup filtered water
- 0.25 cup apple cider vinegar

Directions:

1. Preheat a conventional oven to 350 degrees Fahrenheit

2. Begin by cutting the chicken breast in half to make 2 smaller pieces of meat. Make sure to remove any visible fat at this time.

3. Wrap each piece of meat in a thick plastic wrap.

4. Using a meat cleaver, pound the chicken breasts to make them thinner. This ensures that the meat will cook more evenly and a bit quicker. Set it aside for later.

5. Remove the husk from the garlic and mince it well. Place into a small bowl.

6. In the same small bowl, join the pepper and salt with the minced garlic and rosemary. This will make a rub that you will use on the chicken.

7. Divide the mixed spices into two parts and rub each chicken breast thoroughly with each portion of the spices.

8. Lay the chicken out flat and place 5-6 spinach leaves on the side facing up of both the chicken breasts.

9. Make a roll out of the chicken and spinach, making sure to roll the chicken tightly. Hold the chicken in place with a toothpick.

10. Place the chicken into an oven-safe baking dish. Add the filtered water and apple cider vinegar to the dish, but don't pour it over the chicken.

11. Bake for 15-17 minutes ensuring chicken is thoroughly cooked before removing it from the oven.

12. Serve immediately.

Strawberry Crepes

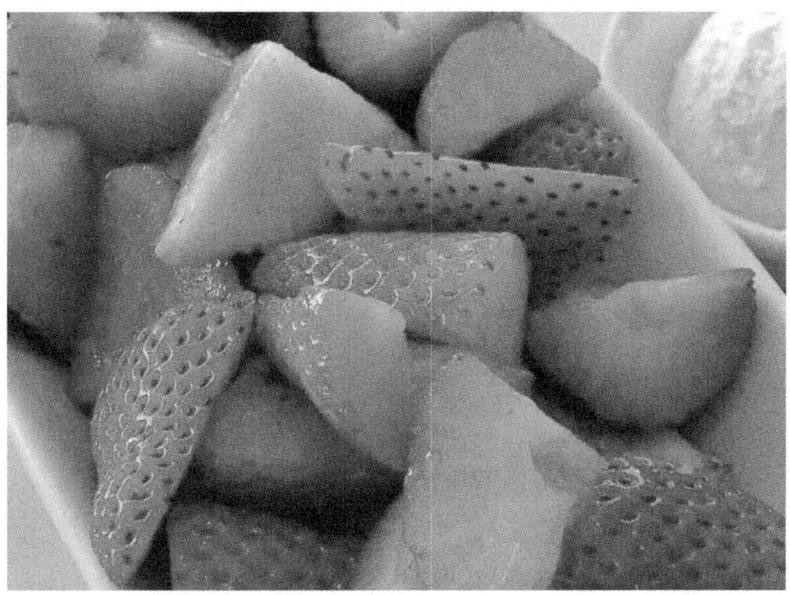

On a lazy weekend morning you can whip up some of these elegant Strawberry Crepes. Can have these crepes at any time.

Time: 25 minutes

Serves: 1

Ingredients:

- 4 large eggs
- 0.25 teaspoon vanilla extract
- 1 tablespoon milk
- 1 tablespoon sugar substitute
- 10 strawberries

Directions:

1. Prepare the strawberries by washing them and cut off their stems.

2. Transfer the strawberries to a cutting board and chop the strawberries into small pieces.

3. Transfer half of the cut strawberries to a small bowl and using a mashing tool, smash the strawberries.

4. Pour the mashed strawberries into a small sauce pan. Add 0.5 tablespoon sugar substitute and cook for 5 minutes, making sure the mixture is warm before removing it from the burner's heat.

5. Over medium heat place a small frying pan.

6. In the small bowl crack one of the eggs and Set it aside for later.

7. In the other small bowl, crack the remaining 3 eggs. With either a slotted spoon or another appropriate tool, take out the 3 yolks and discard them.

8. Add the first egg into the bowl with the three egg whites.

9. Add 1 tablespoon milk, 0.5 tablespoon sugar substitute, and the vanilla extract. Whisk the eggs, milk, and sugar together with the vanilla. You will want the entire egg mixture to appear frothy.

10. Add the egg mixture into a frying pan. Then cook for about 2 min. Wait for the edges of omelet to begin turning light brown before moving onto the next step.

11. After the omelet starts getting brown, use a spatula to carefully flip it onto its other side. Cook for an additional 2 minutes on both sides.

12. Place the cooked eggs on a plate and using the remaining, not mashed strawberry slices, fill the middle of the cooked eggs.

13. Roll the sliced strawberries into the eggs.

14. Poor the mashed warm strawberries over the top of the eggs and serve immediately.

Conclusion

Thank for making it to the end of Simple HCG Cookbook for Beginners. We hope it was informative and able to provide you with all of the tools you need to achieve your weight-loss goals. Remember, sticking to a diet can be hard work, but if you follow these recipes, success will be easier to attain. Each pound lost is a small victory!

If you found this book useful in any way, a review on Amazon is always appreciated! Good luck on your personal weight-loss journey!

About the Author

Born in New Germantown, Pennsylvania, Stephanie Sharp received a Masters degree from Penn State in English Literature. Driven by her passion to create culinary masterpieces, she applied and was accepted to The International Culinary School of the Art Institute where she excelled in French cuisine. She has married her cooking skills with an aptitude for business by opening her own small cooking school where she teaches students of all ages.

Stephanie's talents extend to being an author as well and she has written over 400 e-books on the art of cooking and baking that include her most popular recipes.

Sharp has been fortunate enough to raise a family near her hometown in Pennsylvania where she, her husband and children live in a beautiful rustic house on an extensive piece of land. Her other passion is taking care of the furry members of her family which include 3 cats, 2 dogs and a potbelly pig named Wilbur.

Watch for more amazing books by Stephanie Sharp coming out in the next few months.

Author's Afterthoughts

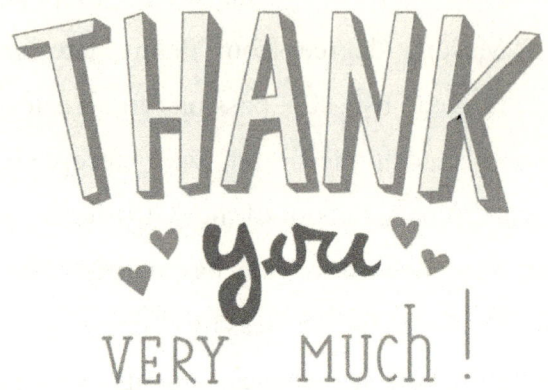

I am truly grateful to you for taking the time to read my book. I cherish all of my readers! Thanks ever so much to each of my cherished readers for investing the time to read this book!

With so many options available to you, your choice to buy my book is an honour, so my heartfelt thanks at reading it from beginning to end!

I value your feedback, so please take a moment to submit an honest and open review on Amazon so I can get valuable insight into my readers' opinions and others can benefit from your experience.

Thank you for taking the time to review!

Stephanie Sharp

For announcements about new releases, please follow my author page on Amazon.com!

You can find that at:

https://www.amazon.com/author/stephanie-sharp

*or Scan **QR-code** below.*

Made in the USA
Las Vegas, NV
01 August 2021